DISCOVER THE HEALING SECRETS OF TURMERIC (GUIDE)

DR. ALICE ONOFUA

Copyright © 2019 by **DR. ALICE ONOFUA**

All rights reserved. Printed in the United States of America. No part of this book may be used or reproduced in any manner whatsoever without written permission except in the case of brief quotations embodied in critical articles or reviews.

TABLE OF CONTENTS

INTRODUCTION 4
CHAPTER ONE 6
   WHAT IS TURMERIC? 6
      History of turmeric 7
   RESOURCES FIND IN TURMERIC 9
CHAPTER TWO 10
   HEALTH BENEFITS OF TURMERIC 10
CHAPTER THREE 20
   FAST FACTS ON TURMERIC 20
CHAPTER FOUR 22
   SIDE EFFECTS OF TURMERIC 222
   FREQUENTLY ASKED QUESTIONS ABOUT TURMERIC 25
ABOUT THE AUTHOR 34
ACKNOWLEDGMENTS 35

Introduction

One of the gifts of nature to mankind is a plant called Turmeric. This plant is richly blessed for it has many healing effects more than we know or appreciate.

Turmeric in India is known as "India Safron". It is an important commercial spice crop grown in India. It is used in diversified form as a condiment, flavouring and colouring agent and as a principal ingredient culinary as curry powder. It has anti-cancer and anti-viral activities; hence finds use not in the drug industry only but cosmetics industry as well.

Turmeric is the dried rhizome of curcuma longa – an herbaceous perennial belonging to the family of Zingiberaceae.
Turmeric's underground stems (rhizomes) are dried and made into capsules, tablets, teas, or extracts and powder which are also made into paste for skin conditions.

Turmeric contains Bioactive Compounds with powerful medicinal properties.

Turmeric contains Curcuminoids and Curcumin. What is Curcumin and its scientifically proven health benefits?

Studies show that Turmeric is the most effective nutritional supplement in existence for ages.

The global production of Turmeric is around 11 lakh tons per annum thereby underlining its importance, marketability (Imports/Exports potentials) and uses.

Want to stay healthy? Want to age with Grace? Want to spend little and achieve optimal result? If yes, you need to discover the secrets hidden in this plant called Turmeric.

Chapter One

WHAT IS TURMERIC?

Turmeric is a popular spice that contains curcumin: A powerful bioactive coumpound. The plant is propagated form rhizomes. The leaves are long, broad and bright green. The flowers are pale yellow and home on dense spikes. The pseudostems are shorter than leaves. The rhizomes are needy for harvesting in about 7-9 months after planting. However, it requires a conversion period of two years.

Turmeric sometimes called Indian saffron or the golden spice; it is a plant that grows mainly in Asia and Central America. It has warm bitter taste.

History of turmeric

For hundreds of years, people around the world have been using Turmeric for its healing properties and cosmetic benefits. It has been used for centuries in traditional India and Chinese medicine. Today, it is go-to for stomach and bowel problems, arthritis.

India is the largest producer, consumer and exporter of Turmeric. Other major producers of Turmeric are Thailand, South East, Asian countries, Central and Latin America and Taiwan.

The global production of Turmeric is around 11 lakh tons per annum. India dominates the world production scenario contributing 78% followed by China 8% myanamr 4% and Nigeria and Bangladesh together contributing 6%.

India is the global leader in value added products of Turmeric and exports. Other major exporters are Thailand, South East Asian Countries, Central and Latin America and Taiwan.
United Arab emirate (UAE) is the major importer of Turmeric from India accounting for 18%, of the total exports followed by United States of America 8%.

The other leading importers are Bangladesh, Japan and Sri Lanka, United Kingdom, Malaysia, South Africa, Netherland and Saudi Arabia – All these Countries accounted for 75% of the world imports and Asian Countries are the main suppliers to the entire world.

The remaining 25% is met by Europe, North America, Central and Latin America Countries.

United States of America imports 97% of its Turmeric requirements from India and remaining portion from the Islands of the Pacific and Thailand. Out of the total global production United Arab Emirates accounts for 18% of the imports followed by United States of America 11%, Japan 9%, Sri Lanka, United Kingdom, Malaysia together accounting for 17%.

Types of turmeric

There are two dominant types of Turmeric found in the world markets:
Madras
Allepey
Both named after the regions of production in India.

Madras Turmeric is preferred by the British and Middle Eastern markets for its more intense brighter and lighter yellow colour.

The orange-yellow flesh Allepey Turmeric is predominantly imported by the United States of America where users prefer it as a spice and a food colourant. It contains about 3.5% to 5.5% volatile oils and 4.0% to 7.0% curcumin

Resources find in turmeric

Turmeric contains curcuminoids and curcumin.
Curcumin is the main active ingredients and has powerful inflammatory effects and is a strong antioxidant and may also help improve symptoms of depression and arthritis. However, the Curcumin content is around 3%.

Curcumin is a remarkably powerful antioxidant, helping to fight oxidative damage and boosting the body's own antioxidant enzymes. This is important because oxidative damage is believed to be one of the key mechanisms behind ageing and many diseases.
Turmeric's underground stems (rhizomes) are dried and made into capsules, tablets, teas, or extracts and Turmeric powder is also made into paste for skin conditions.

Turmeric is the dried rhizome of Curcuma longa – an herbaceous perennial belonging to the family of zingiberaceae.

Turmeric in India is known as "India Safron". It is an important commercial spice crop grown in India. It is used in diversified form as a condiment, flavouring and colouring agent and as a principal ingredient in India culinary as curry powder. It has anti-cancer and anti-viral activities and hence finds use in the drug industry and cosmetics industry.

Chapter Two

Health benefits of turmeric

Turmeric and especially its most active compound curcumin have many scientifically proven health benefits as highlighted below:

TURMERIC CONTAINS BIOACTIVE COMPOUNDS WITH POWERFUL MEDICINAL PROPERTIES

Turmeric contains compounds with medicinal properties called **curcuminoids** and *curcumin* the most important because it is the main active ingredients. Reason being that it has powerful anti inflammatory effect and is a strong antioxidant.

ANTI-INFLAMMATORY COMPOUND

Inflammation is incredibly important because without it, pathogens like bacteria could easily destroy the body or kill. Curcumin helps the body fight foreign invaders and also play a significant role in repairing damage. Although acute, short term inflammation is beneficial, it can become a major problem when it becomes chronic and inappropriately attacks tissues in the body.

Scientists believe that chronic low level inflammation plays a major role in almost every chronic, Western disease. These include heart disease, cancer metabolic syndrome, Alzheimer's and various degenerative conditions. Therefore, anything that can help fight chronic inflammation is of potential importance in preventing and even treating these diseases. Its bioactive substance fights inflammation at the molecular level. Although acute, short inflammation is beneficial, it can become a major problem when it becomes chronic and inappropriately attacks tissues in the body. It blocks NF-KB, a molecule that travels into the nuclei of body cells and turns on genes related to inflammation. NF-KB is believed to play a major role in many chronic diseases.

CURCUMIN DRAMATICALLY INCREASES THE ANTIOXIDANT CAPACITY OF THE BODY

Oxidative damage is believed to be one of the mechanisms behind aging and many diseases. It involves free radicals, highly reactive molecules with unpaired electrons. Free radicals tend to react with important organic substances such as fatty acids, proteins in DNA. That is why antioxidant are so beneficial, reason being that they protect the body from free radicals.

Curcumins comes in again as a potent antioxidant that can neutralize free radicals due to its chemical structure. Moreover, curcumin boosts the activity of the body's antioxidant enzymes. By so doing, delivers a one-two punch against free radicals.

Firstly it blocks them directly and secondly stimulates body's antioxidant defenses.

TURMERIC IMPROVED BRAIN FUNCTION AND A LOWER RISK OF BRAIN DISEASES

Before, it was believed that neurons weren't able to divide and multiply after early childhood. However, it's now known that this does happen.

Neurons are capable of forming new connections, but in certain areas of the brain they can also multiply and increase in number. One of the main drivers of this process is Brain-derived Neurotrophic Factor (BDNF) which is a type of growth hormone that functions in the brain. Many common brain disorders have been linked to decreased levels of this hormone including depression and Alzheimer's disease.

Interestingly, curcumin can increase brain levels of Brain-derived Neurotrophic Factor (BDNF). By doing so, it may be effective in delaying or even reversing many brain diseases and age related decreases in brain function. Curcumin boosts levels of the brain hormone BDNF, which increases the growth of new neurons and fights various degenerative processes in the brain.

CURCUMIN LOWERS RISK OF HEART DISEASE

Over many decades, researches have shown that heart disease is the number one cause or death in the world. It is not surprising that heart disease is incredibly complicated and various things are responsible for this. Interestingly too, curcumin may help reverse many steps in the heart disease process.

Studies have shown that the main benefit of curcumin when it comes to heart disease is by improving the function of the endothelium: the lining of the blood vessel. Endothelial dysfunction is a major driver of heart disease and involves an inability of the endothelium to regulate blood pressure, blood clotting and various other factors. Several studies suggest that curcumin leads to improvements in endothelial function.

For instance, one study found that it's as effective as exercise while another shows that it works as well as the drug ATORVASTATIN.

Moreover, curcumin reduces inflammation and oxidation which play a role in heart disease as well.

One study randomly assigned 121 people, who were undergoing coronary artery bypass surgery either a placebo or 4 grams of curcumin per day a few days before and after surgery. The curcumin group had a 65% decreased risk of experiencing a heart attack in the hospital. In short, curcumin has beneficial effects on several factors known to play a role in the heart disease. It improves the function of the endothelium and is a potent anti-inflammatory agent and antioxidant.

TURMERIC CAN HELP PREVENT AND PERHAPS EVEN TREAT CANCER

Cancer is a terrible disease: characterized by uncontrolled cell growth. There are different forms of Cancer which still have several things in common. Some of them appear to be affected by curcumin supplement.

Studies have proved curcumin to be a beneficial herb in Cancer treatment and found to affect Cancer growth, development and spread at the molecular level.

Furthermore, studies have shown that it can contribute to the death of cancerous cells and reduce angiogenesis (growth of new blood vessels in tumors) and Meta stasis (spread of Cancer)

Multiple studies indicate that curcumin can reduce the growth of cancerous cells in the laboratory and inhibit the growth of tumors in test animals.

However, whether high dose curcumin (preferably with an absorption enhancer like piperine) can help treat Cancer in humans is yet to be studied properly. That notwithstanding, there is evidence that it may prevent Cancer from occurring in the first place especially Cancers of the digestive system like colorectal Cancer.

In a 30-day study in 44 men with lesion in the colon that sometimes turn cancerous, 4 grams of Curcumin per day reduced the number of lesions by 40%.

Curcumin leads to several changes on the molecular level that may help prevent and perhaps even treat Cancer.

CURCUMIN MAY BE USEFUL IN PREVENTING AND TREATING ALZHEIMER'S DISEASE

Alzheimer's disease is a progressive disorder that causes brain cells to waste away (degenerate) and dies. That is,

Alzheimer's disease is the most common cause of dementia – a continuous decline in thinking, behavioral and social skills that disrupts a person's ability to function independently.

Having said that Alzheimer's disease is the most common neurodegenerative disease in the world and a leading cause of dementia, it is rather unfortunate that no good treatment is available for the disease yet. Therefore, preventing it from occurring in the first place is of utmost importance. There may be hope on the horizon because curcumin has been shown to cross the blood brain disease barrier. It is known that inflammation and oxidative damage play a role in Alzheimer's disease and curcumin has beneficial effects in both.

In addition, a key feature of Alzheimer's disease is a build up of protein tangles called amyloid plaques. Studies show that curcumin can help clear these plaques. Curcumin can cross the blood brain barrier and has been showed to lead to various improvements in the pathological process of Alzheimer's disease.

CURCUMIN SUPPLEMENTS HELPS ARTHRITIS

Arthritis is a common problem in Western countries. It is a common disorder characterized by joint inflammation. It can affect one joint or multiple joints. There are more than 100 different types of arthritis, with different causes and treatment methods. Two of the most common types are osteoarthritis (OA) and rheumathoid arthritis (RA).

Studies show that arthritis patients respond very well to curcumin supplements. It helps treat symptoms of arthritis and in some cases more effective than anti-inflammation drugs. For instance, in a study people with rheumatoid arthritis, curcumin was even more effective than an anti- inflammatory drug.

Moreover, many other studies have looked at the effects of curcumin in arthritis and noted improvement in various symptoms.

The Arthritis foundation cites several studies in which Turmeric has reduced inflammation.
This anti-inflammatory ability might reduce the aggravation that people with arthritis feel in their joints.
The Foundation suggests taking Turmeric capsules of 400 – 600 mg up to three times daily for inflammation relief.

TURMERIC RELIEVES PAINS

Studies seem to support Turmeric for pain relief. With one study noting that it seemed to work as well as Ibuprofen (Advil) in people with Arthritis in their knees. Though dosing recommendations seem to vary, those who participated in the Study took 800 mg of Turmeric in capsule form each day.

CURCUMIN HELPS AGAINST DEPRESSION

WHAT IS DEPRESSION?

A mental condition characterized by feelings or severe despondency and dejection, typically also with feelings of inadequacy and guilt, often accompanied by lack of energy and disturbance of appetite and sleep.

Curcumin has shown some promise in treating depression. What is the proof? In a controlled trial, 60 people with depression were randomized into three groups: one group took Prozac; another group took 1gram of Curcumin while the third group took both Prozac and curcumin. After 6 weeks, curcumin had led to improvements that were similar to Prozac's. The group that took both Prozac and curcumin fared better. Which means curcumin was as effective as Prozac in alleviating symptoms of the condition.
According to a study, curcumin is as effective as an antidespressant.

Depression is also linked to reduced levels of brain-derived neurotrophic factor (BDNF) and shrinking hippocampus, a brain area with a role in learning and memory.
Curcumin boosts BDNF levels, potentially reversing some of those changes. There is also some evidence that curcumin can boost the brain neurotransmitters serotonin and dopamine.

HELPS DIGESTION:

Turmeric adds flavor to food, which explains its presence in curry powder. However, it can also play an important role in digesting food. The spice can contribute to healthy digestion as a result of its antioxidant and anti-inflammatory properties.

Turmeric is used in ayurvedic medicine as a digestive healing agent. Western medicine has now begun to study how Turmeric can help with gut inflammation and gut permeability: two measures of digestive efficiency. The spice is even being explored as a treatment for irritable bowel syndrome (IBS).

CURCUMIN MAY HELP DELAY AGEING AND FIGHT AGE RELATED CHRONIC DISEASES

It is generally believed that if curcumin can really help prevent heart disease, cancer and Alzheimer's, it would have obvious benefits for longevity. For this reason, curcumin has become very popular as an anti-aging supplement.
Given the fact that oxidation and inflammation are believed to play a role in aging, Curcumin may have effect that goes beyond just preventing disease.

IMPROVES LIVER FUNCTION:

The liver is a large, meaty organ that sits on the right side of the belly. The liver also detoxifies chemicals and metabolizes drugs. As it does so, the liver secretes bile that ends up back in the intestines. The liver also makes protein important for the blood clotting and other functions.

The antioxidant effect of Turmeric appears to be so powerful that it may stop liver from being damaged by toxins.
This could be good news for people who take strong drugs for diabetics or other health conditions that might hurt their liver with long term use.

Chapter Three

Fast facts on turmeric

Climate and soil Turmeric requires a warm and humid climate. It can be grown in diverse tropical conditions from sea level to 1500mm above MSL with a temperature range 20-30c with a rainfall of 1500mm or more per annum or under irrigated conditions.

Though Turmeric thrives in different types of soil ranging from light black loam, red soil to clayey loams, rich loamy soils having natural drainage and irrigation facilities are the best. Turmeric cannot stand water stagnation or alkalinity. Turmeric can be cultivated organically as an intercrop along with other crops provided that all the companion crops are also organically grown. In some area, Turmeric is grown as an intercrop with mango, jack and litchi and on the West Coast with coconut and areca nut.

Turmeric may be the most effective nutitional supplement in existence.
Many high quality studies show that it has major benefits for body and brain.

Turmeric is the spice that gives curry its yellow colour

Turmeric has been used in India for thousands of years as a spice and medicinal herb.

Most of the Studies on the herb are using Turmeric extracts that contain mostly Curcumin itself with dosage usually exceeding 1gram per day. Using only the Turmeric spice in foods may not be adequate enough to reach the required level, except one takes supplement that contains significant amount of Curcumin. Unfortunately though, Curcumin is poorly absorbed into the bloodstream. It significantly helps taking it with black pepper which contains piperine – a natural substance that enhances the absorption of Curcumin by 2,000%.

The best Curcumin supplement contains piperine which substantially increases the effectiveness.

Turmeric is also fat soluble, therefore, it will be ideal to take it with fatty meal.

Turmeric and especially its most active compound - Curcumin have many scientifically proven health benefits, such as the potential to prevent heart disease, Alzheimer's and Cancer.

Turmeric is used for condition involving pains and inflammation such as osteoarthritis. It is used for hay fever, depression, high cholesterol, liver disease and itching. Moreover, it is used for heartburns, thinking and memory skill, inflammatory bowel disease, stress and many other conditions.

Chapter Four

Side effects of turmeric

While Turmeric does provide potential health benefits, it creates some risks that are worth considering before consuming large amounts.

1. STOMACH UPSET

The same agents in Turmeric that supports digestive health can irritate when taken in large amounts. Some participants in studies looking at the use of Turmeric for Cancer treatment had to drop out because then digestion was so negatively affected.
Turmeric stimulates the stomach to produce more gastric acid while this helps some people's digestion, it can negatively affect others.

2. BLOOD THINNING PROPERTIES

The purifying properties of Turmeric may also lead to bleeding more easily. The reason for this is unclear. Other suggested benefits, such as lowered cholesterol and lowered blood pressure might have something to do with the way Turmeric functions in the blood. People who take blood thinning drugs, such as warfarin (Coumadin) should avoid consuming large doses of Turmeric.

3. STIMULATING CONTRACTIONS

Pregnant women should avoid taking Turmeric supplements because of its blood thinning effects. Adding small amounts of Turmeric to food as spice should not cause health problems.

4. GASTROINTESTINAL PROBLEMS

Turmeric in amounts tested for health purposes is generally considered safe when taken by mouth or applied to the skin. However, high doses or long term use of Turmeric may cause gastrointestinal problems.

RISK FACTORS OF TURMERIC

Do not use Turmeric if you have gallstones or a bile duct obstruction. Bleeding problems: Taking turmeric might slow blood clotting. This might increase the risk of bruising and bleeding in people with bleeding disorders:

Curcumin, a chemical in Turmeric, might decrease blood sugar in people with diabetes.

HOW DOES TURMERIC WORK?

Turmeric contains Bioactive Compounds with powerful Medicinal Properties. Turmeric is the spice that gives curry its yellow color.

Curcumin is the main active ingredient in turmeric. It has powerful anti-inflammatory effects and is a very strong antioxidant.

For anti-inflammatory effects, one needs to get 500 to 1,000 milligrams of curcuminoids per day. When using the spice on its own, the common rule of thumb is that there are 200 milligrams of curcumin in one teaspoon of fresh or ground Turmeric (though it varies a bit depending on the source and origins).

The best time to take curcumin is three or more hours before or after eating a meal; in other words, after fasting. This is when curcumin absorption will be higher.

The primary antioxidant present in turmeric is curcumin. Though having huge quantities of Turmeric is surely not a way to lose weight, but turmeric is said to reduce the inflammation associated with obesity. Thus,
it can give weight loss plan a boost.

PRECAUTIONS

Can Turmeric capsules be taken on empty stomach? One may ask.
The simple answer is that it depends on the condition of the user. Taking 400-800mg of a curcumin supplement on an empty stomach (30 minutes before a meal or two hours after one) is recommended. However, where one experiences heartburn, one can simply take it with food.

FREQUENTLY ASKED QUESTIONS ABOUT TURMERIC

(1) What is turmeric?

Turmeric's scientific name is curcuma longa. It's a rhizome, an underground stem, of a plant that's in the ginger family. It's native to India and Southeast Asia, and it's been used by people of these regions for thousands of years as a food and as a medicine. It can be consumed fresh—in India, this is usually in a pickled form, or as a powder. It can also be juiced. It's called haridrā in Sanskrit, haldī in Hindi, and halad in Marathi, to give you a few of its native names.

(2) What are its traditional uses in India?

In Ayurvedic medicine, turmeric is used:

- Topically for a variety of skin conditions, including

skin infections.

- To improve the skin's appearance. In traditional Indian weddings, both the bride and the groom apply a paste of Turmeric, mixed along with other ingredients such as sandalwood, onto their skin to enhance the skin's glow.

- As a food coloring and flavoring agent.

- For coughs and colds.

- As an antiparasitic medication.

- As an anti-itch medicine.

- As a medicine to treat Type II Diabetes, urinary tract infections, gout, and even haemorrhoids.

- As a regulator of the immune system, as a liver tonic, and even as a hair remover.

- As a dye for fabrics.

Turmeric has always been used in Hindu ceremonies. It's very much a part of the everyday culture. You can't have India without Turmeric.

In Ayurveda, it's always preferred to take any as a food. Turmeric is no exception. It's used in cooking and you only need a little bit.

With all of its amazing traditional uses, it caught the eye of scientists who wanted to study it and figure out why it was such a magical spice.

(3) What is curcumin?

What's the difference between curcumin and Turmeric? Aren't they the same thing?

They're not. Curcumin is just one chemical isolated or extracted from Turmeric, and it gives Turmeric its characteristic yellow color. It belongs to a larger family of chemicals called curcuminoids. Since its discovery, it's been glorified as a miracle compound. I'll use a cliche here—turmeric is greater than the sum of its parts. We still don't know all the different chemicals that it contains. Curcumin is only one small chemical component of the Turmeric rhizome. So therefore, Turmeric should be consumed as whole food so we don't miss out on other important compounds that may not have yet been discovered by modern science. Just like, proverbially, we eat an apple a day to keep the Doctor away, right? Nobody ever said, "A capsule of malic acid," or "a tablet of farnesene keeps the Doctor away." Just because these chemicals are key components of apples, we don't equate them with the WHOLE fruit. We don't swallow capsules filled with these chemicals as apple substitutes.

You may remember the hype around beta-carotene in the 1990s. It's a chemical that can be found in food such as carrots. It was quite a celebrated supplement in its heyday until a couple of studies showed that it may increase the risk of lung cancer in smokers. It lost its sexy status almost overnight. But you and I know, using our common sense, which whole foods containing beta carotene are not going to hurt you, unless of course, you overdose on them. And it does happen—people can literally turn ORANGE. This is a condition called carotenemia or carotenosis.

(4) How is curcumin taken, and how is it dosed? AND

(5) How is turmeric taken and how is it dosed?

You generally buy curcumin in tablet or capsule form. The same goes for turmeric.

The strengths and dosages are really high; in fact they're very high. 500mg of curcumin twice daily is a common dose, while 1500 mg of Turmeric three times daily is a common dose. This is really over-the-top. Sometimes I feel in the supplement industry, the motto is "go big or go home." Why is it so hard to imagine that food can be medicine? Is that too simplistic? Is it not trendy enough? Recently there was a reported case about a Doctor who administered a Turmeric emulsion intravenously to a woman, causing her to lose her life. There is such a thing as too much of a good thing!

(6) What are curcumin's side effects?

Curcumin supplements MAY slow down blood clotting, so if you must take curcumin, your Doctor may have you stop it a couple of weeks before a scheduled surgery. It may also interact with anticoagulant and antiplatelet drugs. Bottom line: If you're taking it, please tell your Doctor you're on it. He or she will appreciate it.

Curcumin, IN ISOLATION is considered an estrogen-like compound; so this can, in theory, in the megadoses consumed, worsen hormone-sensitive conditions such as certain breast/uterine/ovarian cancers. In theory, it may also affect sperm count. Realistically, though, look at the population of India where close to 100% of the population ingests Turmeric which contains curcumin. Why does the country overall (not talking about individual cases of infertility here) seem to NOT have a male fertility problem? It is probably because nobody is popping curcumin capsules in India. They don't now, nor did they ever. People are not ingesting megadoses of isolated curcumin which of course can be expected to have side effects.

(7) So if curcumin's no good, is it better then, to take turmeric capsules?

The answer again is "No." Because again, this this is a reductionist approach, much like taking curcumin. It's an oversimplified solution, and not a good one. If one have a problem, say knee pain, then a turmeric supplement—just because turmeric contains anti-inflammatory compounds— isn't going to magically fix it. The first thing to do would be to look at other things first, such as modest weight loss or exercise, or changing one's diet. Taking high doses of supplements cannot cancel out years of an unhealthy lifestyle or diet.

Besides this, let's consider other reasons why this is not a good medical practice, from a Western medical standpoint or an Ayurvedic medical standpoint.

First of all, 1 gram of turmeric powder measures out to be almost 1/2 a teaspoon. So if you're taking 1500mg three times a day, you're taking about 2 to 2.25 teaspoons of raw turmeric powder a day. Imagine taking that much raw turmeric powder every day for years? Something bad is bound to happen. Because the powder is ALREADY a concentrated (dehydrated) version of the root! If turmeric powder is about 2% curcumin by weight, how many of those rhizomes are you eating when you take a curcumin supplement? Even as an Ayurvedic supplement in India, most people do not ingest more than 1 teaspoon of turmeric powder a day. If they take turmeric as a supplement, it's generally mixed into milk or another oily vehicle and it's taken for a short period of time. It's a powerful medicine. Therefore you need very little. Much like you don't use a steamroller to fold a piece of origami paper, you don't need such a large daily dose of turmeric.

Another disadvantage from an Ayurvedic point of view is that a capsule will bypass the tongue. Turmeric needs to physically come in contact with the tongue and saliva. When we taste it and recognize it as food that's when digestion truly begins to take place. We all know that digestion actually starts when we smell, or look at, or even think of food, because these sensations send messages to our brain which in turn sends messages to get our saliva and other digestive juices flowing. A capsule would bypass this first critical phase of digestion.

(8) How should turmeric be consumed if not in pill form?

Properties of Haldi per the Ayurveda texts are: bitter, pungent, drying (ruksha), light (laghu) and hot (ushna). When cooking it, to balance these properties we have to use substances with opposite qualities. And therefore, Turmeric is never used alone in Indian dishes; it is always combined with other spices such as cumin, coriander, and fennel. Also, a fat has to be involved in the cooking process, because Turmeric has molecules that are fat-soluble as well as water-soluble. So we heat Turmeric in a fat such as oil or ghee. Or, we heat it in milk because not only is milk a fatty substance, but *because it is* considered a cooling substance. So you can see how in a capsule form or by simply adding Turmeric powder to water, we're going to get less bioavailability. When the drug isn't used properly by the body, we run into side effects. This is why adding Turmeric powder or Turmeric root (if you're trying to embrace the whole food philosophy) to ice-cold predominantly water-based smoothies is a bad idea. To sum it up, Turmeric has to be (a) physically heated—even though it is considered a "hot" spice (b) heated in an oil or fat and (c) balanced out with other "cooling" spices. The Ayurvedic concept of hot and cool foods will be taken up in another post, hopefully soon.

(9) Why are large doses of turmeric or curcumin put into those capsules?

This is because Turmeric and curcumin have poor bioavailability—when they are not cooked properly, like I just talked about in question number 8. So to fix this, black pepper is often added to the capsule to enhance bioavailability. Well, now we have another problem on our hands! According to Ayurveda, black pepper is considered another hot and pungent substance. With the additive effect of two similarly heating spices you run into problems such as gastroesophageal reflux, heartburn, worsening peptic ulcers. The supplement may even drop your blood sugar.

CONSUMER INFORMATION USE

This book is just a guide on the health benefits of Turmeic. It is not a specific medical advice intended to replace information or advice from your medical personnel. It is only your healthcare provider that fully understands your health challenges and as such, has the knowledge and requisite training to provide the right and necessary medical advice for you.

In essence, you should not rely on the information provided by this guide to decide whether or not to use or accept your medical personnel's advice regarding the use of any natural products or similar treatments, therapies or life-style choices.

Please also note that this book does not recommend or endorse any natural products or similar treatments, therapies or life-style choices as safe, effective or approved for treating any health condition whatsoever.

Furthermore, this book does not encapsulates all information about natural products, possible uses, directions, warnings, precautions, interactions, advserse effects or riks applicable to you. You are advised to consult your medical personnel for complete information about your heath status and available or recommended treatment options.

About the Author

Dr. Alice Onofua is a Professor of bology at the University of California. She received her M.D in penn state and eventually earned her spot at Pennsylvania hospital in the emergency center. She has devoted much of her life to the study of human anatomy and physiology, and has pioneered early learning research through Anatomy Education Research Institute (AERI). Dr. Alice is also a publisher. Her articles on different subjects about how body system can grow naturally without the effect of using drugs or checking medical centers have appeared in leading professional publications and her work has been profiled in hundreds of other media reports.

Acknowledgments

My appreciation goes to God Almighty for the opportunity and wisdom he gave me to complete this book.

Profound thanks to those whose materials, writings, research work or advice contributed one way or the other to the success of this book.

THANKS FOR READING

www.ingramcontent.com/pod-product-compliance
Lightning Source LLC
Chambersburg PA
CBHW070906220526
45466CB00005B/2143